The REAL BIG Weight Loss

Works for everyone.

All the time!

1st edition - August, 2018

Eat less!

Eat less!

Eat less!

Eat less!

Eat less!

Eat less!

Eat less!

Eat less!

Eat less!

Eat less!

Eat less!

Eat less!

Eat less!

Eat less!

Eat less!

Eat less!

Eat less!

Eat less!

Eat less!

Eat less!

Eat less!

Eat less!

Eat less!

Eat less!

Eat less!

Eat less!

Eat less!

Eat less!

Eat less!

Eat less!

Eat less!

Eat less!

Eat less!

Eat less!

Eat less!

Eat less!

Eat less!

Eat less!

Eat less!

Eat less!

Eat less!

Eat less!

Eat less!

Eat less!

Eat less!

Eat less!

Eat less!

Eat less!

Eat less!

Eat less!

Eat less!

Eat less!

Eat less!

Eat less!

Eat less!

Eat less!

Eat less!

Eat less!

Eat less!

Eat less!

Eat less!

Eat less!

Eat less!

Eat less!

Eat less!

Eat less!

Eat less!

Eat less!

Eat less!

Eat less!

Eat less!

Eat less!

Eat less!

Eat less!

Eat less!

Eat less!

Eat less!

Eat less!

Eat less!

Eat less!

Eat less!

Eat less!

Eat less!

Eat less!

Eat less!

Eat less!

Eat less!

Eat less!

Eat less!

Eat less!

Eat less!

Eat less!

Eat less!

Eat less!

Eat less!

Eat less!

Eat less!

Eat less!

Eat less!

Eat less!

Eat less!

Eat less!

Eat less!

Eat less!

Eat less!

Eat less!

Eat less!

Eat less!

Eat less!

Eat less!

Eat less!

Eat less!

Eat less!

Eat less!

Eat less!

Eat less!

Eat less!

Eat less!

Eat less!

Eat less!

Eat less!

Eat less!

Eat less!

Eat less!

Eat less!

Eat less!

Eat less!

Eat less!

Eat less!

Eat less!

Eat less!

Eat less!

Eat less!

Eat less!

Eat less!

Eat less!

Eat less!

Eat less!

Eat less!

Eat less!

Eat less!

Eat less!

Eat less!

Eat less!

Eat less!

Eat less!

Eat less!

Eat less!

Eat less!

Eat less!

Eat less!

152

Eat less!

Eat less!

Eat less!

Eat less!

Eat less!

Eat less!

Eat less!

Eat less!

Eat less!

Eat less!

Eat less!

Eat less!

Eat less!

Eat less!

Eat less!

Eat less!

Eat less!

Eat less!

Eat less!

Eat less!

Eat less!

Eat less!

Eat less!

Eat less!

Eat less!

Eat less!

Eat less!

Eat less!

Eat less!

www.ingramcontent.com/pod-product-compliance
Lightning Source LLC
Chambersburg PA
CBHW021143260726
48656CB00024B/1391